theory in a
Nutshell

A Guide to
Health Promotion Theory

Don Nutbeam and Elizabeth Harris

The McGraw-Hill Companies, Inc

Sydney   New York   San Francisco   Auckland
Bangkok   Bogotá   Caracas   Hong Kong
Kuala Lumpur   Lisbon   London   Madrid
Mexico City   Milan   New Delhi   San Juan
Seoul   Singapore   Taipei   Toronto

McGraw·Hill Australia

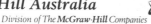

A Division of The McGraw·Hill Companies

National Library of Australia Cataloguing-in-Publication data:

Nutbeam, Don.
Theory in a nutshell : a guide to health promotion theory.

ISBN 0 074 70821 X.

1. Health promotion. 2. Health planning. I. Harris,
Elizabeth. II. Title.

613

Published in Australia by
McGraw-Hill Book Company Australia Pty Limited
4 Barcoo Street, Roseville NSW 2069, Australia
Acquisitions Editor: Meiling Voon
Production Editor: Sybil Kesteven
Cover design: Steve Miller, Miller Hare
Cover image: Miller Hare Design Group
Printed by Hillwing Printing Company, Hong Kong

Contents

List of tables and figures

TABLES

FIGURES

Acknowledgments

Several people have contributed to the development of this monograph. We would particularly like to acknowledge the contribution of Karen Glanz. Her textbook on theory, research and practice is a major resource for students and is referred to regularly in this monograph. Her monograph *Theory at a glance* was the model for this monograph and the inspiration for the title. Karen also provided us with a thoughtful and instructive review of an earlier version of the monograph. Others who have helped us by reviewing earlier drafts are Adrian Bauman, Lesley King, Lyn Stoker and Doug Tutt. Olivia Wroth and Greg Heard of Nullegai Communications edited the final draft.

We would particularly like to thank the NSW Health Department who provided a small seeding grant for the initial research for the monograph, and Kimberly McClean who undertook this initial work.

The purpose of this monograph

Not all health promotion programs are equally successful in achieving their aims and objectives. Experience tells us that programs are most likely to be successful when the determinants of a health problem or issue are well understood, where the needs and motivations of the target population are addressed, and the context in which the program is being implemented has been taken into account. That is, the program 'fits' the problem.

The use of theory can help achieve a better fit between problem and program.

Although many health promotion projects and programs are developed and implemented without overt reference to theory, there is substantial evidence from the literature on health promotion to suggest that the use of theory will significantly improve the chances of success in achieving pre-determined program objectives. The use of theory can help us understand better the nature of the problem being addressed, the needs and motivations of the target population, and/or the context for intervention, thus helping to achieve a better fit between problem and program.

This monograph is intended to provide practitioners and students of health promotion with an overview of several of the most influential theories and models which have guided health promotion practice in the recent past, and remain influential in the present.

In each case, an explanation of the main elements of the theory is provided, followed by a commentary on its relative strengths and weaknesses, and some idea on how it can be related to the real world.

Through this monograph, we hope to demonstrate that, when used prudently, theories can greatly enhance the effectiveness and sustainability of health promotion programs.

Structure of the monograph

This monograph reflects the range of activities that are currently being undertaken by health promotion practitioners. It starts with an examination of theories that explain health behaviour and health behaviour change by focussing on individual characteristics. Four theories that have been influential on health promotion practice are discussed: the health belief model; the theory of reasoned action; the transtheoretical (stages of change) model; and social learning theory.

> Unless behavioral theories are put into the broader context in which the individual is living, many factors that influence health will remain unexplained.

What emerges from these overviews is that while these theories contribute substantially to our understanding of individual behaviour, unless they are put into the broader context in which the individual is living, many factors that influence health will remain unexplained.

It is now well recognised that the capacity and opportunities for individuals to bring about change to their health can be significantly affected by the competence of the community in which they live to address issues beyond the control of any one individual. This means that we need to understand theories and models that help explain how the capacity of communities can be strengthened and how new ideas can best be introduced into communities. Correspondingly, community mobilisation (as reflected in social planning, social action and community development) is discussed as well as the diffusion of innovation theory.

In order to raise awareness and engage individuals, groups and communities in taking action to promote health, a number of theories and models have been developed to guide ways in which health messages can be most effectively communicated and acted upon. The two most influential, communication-behaviour change and social marketing, are discussed. Both have provided very practical and effective guidance to those developing mass communication strategies.

However, their impact is often limited if relevant organisational structures do not support or facilitate the changes they seek to bring about.

Organisational structures (sometimes referred to as settings) can have both direct and indirect impacts on people's health. These settings, such as schools, worksites and recreational venues, are places where people spend a great deal of time. Such settings directly influence health through the services and programs that they provide to individuals and communities, and through the opportunities and constraints they place on individuals and health-related behaviour (e.g. facilities for physical activity, restrictions on smoking). Less directly, such settings influence health by providing access to social support, or more negatively as a source of stress and conflict. They can also have indirect impacts through, for example, planning regulations by councils, and income support polices of the government. In this context this monograph looks at two models that help practitioners to understand how to influence change within organisations and enable them to work effectively together. This are discussed as theories of organisational change and a model for understanding intersectoral action.

Finally this monograph looks at the emerging field of healthy public policy and models that are being developed to understand how policy can be influenced and changed to promote health. These include an ecological framework for policy development, determinants of policy making and indicators of health promotion policy.

TABLE 1: Summary of models presented in the monograph

Area of change	Theories or models
Theories that explain health behaviour and health behaviour change by focussing on the individual	Health belief model Theory of reasoned action Transtheoretical (stages of change) model Social learning theory
Theories that explain change in communities and community action for health	Community mobilisation • Social planning • Social action • Community development Diffusion of innovation
Theories that guide the use of communication strategies for change to promote health	Communication for behaviour change Social marketing
Models that explain changes in organisations and the creation of health-supportive organisational practices	Theories of organisational change Models of intersectoral action
Models that explain the development and implementation of healthy public policy	Ecological framework for policy development Determinants of policy making Indicators of health promotion policy

I. Theory

1.1 What is a theory?

A fully developed theory would be characterised by three major elements. It would explain:

- the major factors that influence the phenomena of interest, for example those factors which explain why some people are regularly active and others are not;
- the relationship between these factors, for example the relationship between knowledge, beliefs, social norms and behaviours such as physical activity; and
- the conditions under which these relationships do or do not occur: the how, when and why of hypothesised relationships, for example, the time, place and circumstances which, predictably, lead to a person being active or inactive.

A commonly used definition of a theory is:

> Systematically organised knowledge applicable in a relatively wide variety of circumstances devised to analyse, predict, or otherwise explain the nature or behaviour of a specified set of phenomena that could be used as the basis for action. [1]

Most health promotion theories come from the behavioural and social sciences. They borrow from various disciplines such as psychology, sociology, management, consumer behaviour and marketing. Such diversity reflects the fact that health promotion practice is not only concerned with the behaviour of individuals but also with the ways in which society is organised and the role of policy and organisational structures in promoting health.

Many of the theories commonly used in health promotion are not highly developed in the way suggested in the definition above, nor have they been rigorously tested when compared, for example, to

[1] Van Ryn M, Heany C A. What's the use of theory? Health Education Quarterly 1992; 19.3: 315–330.a

theory in the physical sciences. They are more accurately referred to as theoretical frameworks or models.

1.2 Linking Theory to program planning

The potential of theory to guide the development of health promotion interventions is substantial. Linking theory to program planning models can assist in developing interventions, predicting issues that may be important and helping to explain difficulties. Program management guidelines for health promotion have also been produced (see further reading at the end of this section for more information). In each case these models and guidelines follow a structured sequence including planning, implementation and evaluation stages. Reference to different theories can guide and inform practitioners at each of these stages.

Figure 1 presents a health promotion planning and evaluation cycle, indicating the various stages in the planning, implementation and evaluation of a health promotion program.

Defining the problem

Identification of the parameters of the health problem to be addressed may involve drawing on a wide range of epidemiological and demographic information, as well as information from the behavioural and social sciences, and knowledge of community needs and priorities. Here, different theories can help us identify what should be the focus for an intervention.

Specifically, theory can inform choice of the elements we should consider as the focus for the intervention. For example, the health belief model, and theory of reasoned action help identify individual characteristics, beliefs and values which are associated with different health behaviours and may be amenable to change. Similarly, organisational change theory helps identify key elements of organisations which may need to be changed and are amenable to change.

FIGURE 1. Health Promotion Planning and Evaluation Cycle

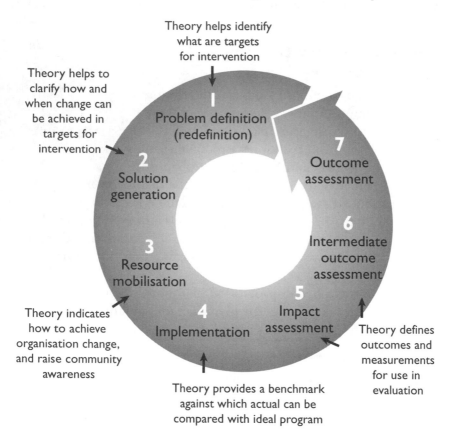

Theory helps identify
what are targets
for intervention

Theory helps to
clarify how and
when change can
be achieved in
targets for
intervention

1 Problem definition
(redefinition)

2 Solution
generation

3 Resource
mobilisation

7 Outcome
assessment

6 Intermediate
outcome
assessment

Theory indicates
how to achieve
organisation change,
and raise community
awareness

4 Implementation

5 Impact
assessment

Theory defines
outcomes and
measurements
for use in
evaluation

Theory provides a benchmark
against which actual can be
compared with ideal program

Planning a solution

The second stage in the cycle indicates the need for the analysis of potential solutions, leading to the development of a program plan which specifies the objectives and strategies to be employed, as well as the sequence of activity. Theory is at its most useful here in providing guidance on how and when change might be achieved in the target population, organisation or policy, and may prompt ideas which would not have routinely occurred to us.

Different theories can help us understand the methods we could use as the focus of our interventions; specifically by improving understanding of the processes by which changes occur in the target variables (i.e. people, organisations and policies), and by clarifying the means of achieving change in these target variables. For example social learning theory helps explain the relationship between personal observation and experience, social norms, and the influence of different external environments on individual behaviour.

Thus, those theories which explain and predict individual and group health behaviour and organisational practice and those which identify methods for changing these determinants of health behaviour and organisational practice are worthy of close consideration in this phase of planning.

Some theories also inform decisions on the timing and sequencing of our interventions in order to achieve maximum effects. For example, stages of change theory and diffusion of innovation theory provide guidance on sequence and timing of activities with individuals and communities respectively.

Mobilising resources for implementation

Once a program plan has been developed, the first phase in implementation is usually directed towards generating public and political interest in the program, mobilising resources for program implementation, and building capacity in partner organisations through which the program may operate (e.g. schools, worksites, local government). The models of intersectoral action which help us understand how to build partnerships, and organisational change theory which indicates how to influence organisational procedures are particularly useful here, as too is communication-behaviour change theory which can guide the development of media-based awareness raising activities.

Implementation

The implementation of a program may involve multiple strategies, such as education and advocacy. Here, the key elements of theory can provide a benchmark against which the actual selection of methods and sequencing of an intervention can be considered in relation to the theoretically ideal implementation of programs.

In this way the use of theory helps us to explain success or failure in different programs, particularly by highlighting the possible impact of differences between planned and actual implementation of the program. It can also assist in identifying the key elements of a program that can form the basis for disseminating successful programs.

Evaluation

Health promotion interventions can be expected to have different levels of impact and different effects over time. Impact evaluation represents the first level of outcome evaluation of a program. The adoption of theory in the planning of programs can provide guidance on the measures which can be used to assess the success of programs. For example where theory suggests that the target of interventions is to achieve change in knowledge and self-efficacy, or changes in social norms or organisational practices, measurement of these changes becomes the first point of evaluation. Such impact measures are often referred to as health promotion outcomes.

Intermediate outcome assessment is the next level of evaluation. Theory can also be used to predict the intermediate health outcomes which are sought from an intervention. Usually these are considered in terms of modification of individual behaviour or modifications to social economic and environmental conditions which determine health or influence behaviour. Several theories, such as the health belief model and social learning theory predict that changes to health promotion outcomes will lead to change in health behaviour.

Health outcome assessment refers to the end-point outcomes of an intervention in terms of change in physical or mental health status, in quality of life, or in improved equity in health within populations. Definition of these final outcomes will be based on theoretically predicted relationships between changes in the determinants of risk (intermediate health outcomes) and final health outcomes.

Figure 1 indicates that each of these evaluation stages leads back to a redefinition of priority problems and solutions; hence the concept of a cycle of planning and evaluation.

Table 2 summarises the tasks and potential of theory to support the planning, execution and evaluation of health promotion programs.

1.3 Single theory or multiple theories?

Theories are not a series of static pronouncements that can be applied to all issues in all circumstances. In health promotion some of the theories that have been used have been extensively refined and developed in the light of experience. The range and focus of theories has also expanded over the past two decades from a concentration on individual behaviour to a concern with seeing the behaviour of individuals as part of a complex web of factors that influence health.

Contemporary health promotion operates at several different levels:
- individual
- community
- organisational settings
- public policy and practice

Choosing the right approach is moderated by the nature of the problem, its determinants and the opportunities for action.

Programs which operate at multiple levels, such as those that draw upon combinations of the strategies described in the Ottawa Charter for Health Promotion, are most likely to address the range of determinants of health problems in populations, and thereby have the greatest effect.

For example, a program to improve uptake of immunisation will generally be more effective when based on a combination of education to inform and motivate individual parents to present their children, facilitation of community debate to change perceptions concerning the safety and convenience of immunisation, changes to organisational practice to improve notification systems, provision of more conveniently located clinics, and financial incentives for parents and doctors.

It follows that no single theory dominates health promotion practice, and nor could it, given the range of health problems and their determinants, the diversity of populations and settings, and differences in available resources and skills among practitioners.

Depending on the level of intervention (individual, group, or organisation), the target of change (simple, one-off behaviour, complex behaviour, organisational or policy change), different theories

> In many cases it will be possible and appropriate to combine different models and theories to achieve goals across the spectrum of health promotion actions.

will have greater relevance, and provide a better fit.

None of the theories or models presented in this monograph can simply be adopted as the answer to all problems. Most often, we benefit by drawing upon more than one of the theories presented here to match the multiple levels of the program response being contemplated.

To be useful and relevant, the different models and theories have to be readily understood, and genuinely capable of application to a wide variety of real-life conditions of practice.

Although we are constantly reminded that 'there is nothing so practical as a good theory', many of us remain somewhat suspicious of the capacity of intervention theories to provide the guidance necessary to develop an effective intervention in a complex environment.

Karen Glanz offers a commonsense summary of how to judge a good fit between a theory or combinations of theories and the problem you are trying to address. It is:

- logical;
- consistent with everyday observations;
- similar to those used in previous successful program examples you have read or heard about; and
- supported by past research in the area or related areas.

While the use of theory alone does not guarantee effective programs, the use of theory in the planning, execution and evaluation of programs will enhance the chances of success. One of the greatest challenges for practitioners is to identify how best to achieve a fit between the issues of interest and established theories or models which could improve the effectiveness of a program or intervention.

This monograph is intended to assist you in meeting this challenge.

Table 2: The use of theory in program planning and evaluation

Planning Phase	Task	Possible use of Theory
Problem identification and prioritisation	Clarify major health issues for a defined population, and prioritise in terms of the potential for effective intervention	Clarify what should be the target elements of an intervention, such as individual beliefs, social norms or organisational practices
Planning a solution	Develop a program plan which specifies program objectives, strategies and the sequence of activity	Guidance on how and when and where change can be achieved in the target elements of a program
Mobilising resources for implementation	Generate public and political support, build the capacity of partner organisations and secure resources	Guidance on how to build partnerships, raise public awareness and foster organisational development
Implementation	Execute the program as planned, utilising multiple strategies (as appropriate to the program objectives)	Provide a benchmark against which the actual implementation can be compared with the theoretically ideal
Evaluation	Assess the impact and outcome of the program according to predefined program objectives	Define outcomes and measurements which could be used at each level of evaluation

Further reading

Glanz K, Lewis FM, Rimer BK. *Health Behaviour and Health Education: Theory, Research and Practice.* San Francisco, CA: Jossey-Bass, 1997.

Green LW, Kreuter MW. *Health Promotion Planning: An Educational and Environmental Approach.* Mountain View, CA: Mayfield, 1991.

Hawe P, Degeling D, Hall J. *Evaluating Health Promotion: A health workers guide.* Sydney: Maclennan and Petty, 1990.

Coppel S. King L, Stoker L, Noort M, Gal S. *Program Management Guidelines for Health Promotion.* Sydney: NSW Health Department, 1994.

2. Theories which explain health behaviour and health behaviour change by focussing on individual characteristics

One of the major roots of contemporary health promotion can be found in the application of health psychology to health behaviour change. Evidence for this can be seen in the phenomenal growth in the discipline of health psychology and the evolution of the concept of behavioural medicine. This discipline has been a significant influence in the USA, where for several decades researchers have sought to explain, predict and change health behaviour by the development and application of theories and models evolving from the disciplines of psychology and the hybrid social-psychology. Four of the most influential are described below.

2.1 The health belief model

The health belief model is one of the longest established theoretical models designed to explain health behaviour by better understanding beliefs about health. It was originally articulated to explain why individuals participate in public health programs such as health checks and immunisation programs, and has been developed for application to other types of health behaviour.

At its core, the model suggests that the likelihood of an individual taking action related to a given health problem is based on the interaction between four different types of belief. Figure 2 summarises the different elements of the model. The model predicts that individuals will take action to protect or promote health if they perceive themselves to be susceptible to a condition or problem, and if they believe it will have potentially serious consequences: the perceived threat. They believe a course of action is available which will reduce their susceptibility, or minimise the consequences, and that the benefits of taking action outweigh the costs or barriers.

Later refinements have acknowledged the important modifying fac-

FIGURE 2: Major elements of the Health Belief Model

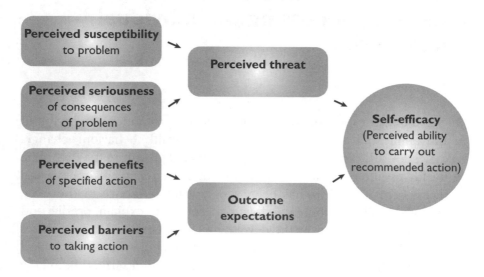

tors, particularly those associated with personal characteristics and social circumstances, and the impact of more immediate cues for action, such as media publicity or personal experience. Added to this analysis is the concept of self-efficacy — that is, the belief in one's competency to take appropriate action — as a further factor influencing the strength of the model in predicting behaviour change.

Thus, for example, if we consider the application of this model to the prevention of Human Immunodeficiency Virus (HIV) infection, in order to adopt behaviours which minimise risk of infection, individuals need to:

- believe that they are at risk of HIV infection;
- believe that the consequences of infection are serious;
- receive supportive cues for action which may trigger a response (such as targeted media publicity);
- believe that risk minimisation practices (such as safe sex or abstinence) will greatly reduce the risk of infection;
- believe that the benefits of action to reduce risk will outweigh

potential costs and barriers, such as reduced enjoyment, and negative reactions of partner and/or community; and,

- believe in their ability to take effective action, such as following and maintaining safe sex practice.

Although it was not always consciously done, many of the early public education campaigns concerning HIV–AIDS prevention conformed to this approach, initially by seeking to persuade people that they are at risk, and by emphasising the deadly nature of Acquired Immune Deficiency Syndrome (AIDS). Later as the epidemic has developed, public education campaigns focussed more on emphasising the efficacy of safe sex (particularly the use of condoms) in minimising the risk of infection, and in improving people's confidence to use condoms.

A 1974 review of findings from interventions using the health belief model provided persuasive evidence to support the usefulness of the model in predicting why individuals adopted (or failed to adopt) different health behaviours. In the twenty years following this publication the model has been widely adopted as a planning tool for health education programs intended to promote greater compliance with preventive health behaviours and health care recommendations.

The health belief model has been found to be most useful when applied to behaviours for which it was originally developed, particularly traditional preventive health behaviours such as immunisation and attendance for health checks, but it was less useful in consideration of long-term, more complex, and socially determined behaviours, such as alcohol and tobacco use.

Overcoming perceived barriers to successful action was identified as the most important element of the model. Perceived susceptibility and perceived benefits were also important.

In a review of the model in 1984 the authors point to the limitations of the health belief model in predicting and explaining health behaviour:

**The health belief model is a psycho-social model;
as such it is limited to accounting for as much of the
variance in an individual's health behaviour as can**

be explained by their attitudes and beliefs. It is clear that other forces influence health actions as well.

These 'other forces' include social, economic and environmental conditions, which significantly shape the barriers to action which are fundamental to the model. For example, limited access to health care services and/or resources can, of course, greatly impede effective health actions, and will in turn influence the individual's perceptions of barriers and benefits which are integral to the model.

If we go back to the example of the HIV–AIDS public education campaigns, some of the limitations of the health belief model become apparent. The lack of accessible sexually transmissible diseases services, the cost or availability of condoms, pressures on some groups (such as commercial sex workers) to act in unsafe ways in order to keep customers, can all work against people adopting behaviours that they know will reduce their risk of infection. Individual behaviour and the beliefs which influence it need to be seen in this wider context.

> Changes in knowledge and beliefs will almost always form part of a comprehensive health promotion program, and the health belief model provides an essential reference point in the development of messages

Commentary

The model's great use is in the relatively simple way in which it illustrates the importance of individual beliefs about health, and beliefs about the relative costs and benefits of actions to protect or improve health. Two decades of research have indicated that promoting change in those beliefs can lead to changes in health behaviour which contribute to improved health status. Changes in knowledge and beliefs will almost always form part of a comprehensive health promotion program, and the health belief model provides a useful reference point in the development of messages to improve knowledge and change beliefs, especially messages designed for use in the print media.

Further reading

Strecher VJ, Rosenstock IM. The Health Belief Model. In: Glanz K et al. *Health Behaviour and Health Education: Theory, Research and Practice.* San Francisco, CA: Jossey-Bass, 1997.

Janz NK, Becker MH. The Health Belief Model: A Decade Later. *Health Education Quarterly 1984*; 11: 1–47.

Harrison JA et al. A meta-analysis of studies of the Health Belief Model. *Health Education Research 1992*; 7.1: 107–116.

2.2 The theories of reasoned action and planned behaviour

The theory of reasoned action was developed by Ajzen and Fishbein to explain human behaviour that is under 'voluntary' control. A major assumption underlying the theory is that people are usually rational and will make predictable decisions in well-defined circumstances. The model is predicated on the assumption that intention to act is the most immediate determinant of behaviour, and that all other factors influencing behaviour will be mediated through behavioural intention.

Figure 3 shows how behavioural intentions are thought to be influenced by attitudes towards behaviours and subjective norms. Attitudes, in this case, are determined by the belief that a desired outcome will occur if a particular behaviour is followed, and that the outcome will be beneficial to health (similar to perceived benefits and barriers in the health belief model).

Subjective norms in this case relate to a person's beliefs about what other people think he or she should do (normative beliefs), and by an individual's motivation to comply with those other people's wishes. These social influences vary in strength related to the degree to which the individual values social approval by a particular group. Thus, for example, if an individual who smokes feels that most people do not smoke and that most of their valued friends and colleagues want them to quit, then it is most likely that the person would consider that there is a norm which favours quitting smoking.

FIGURE 3: Major elements of the Theory of Planned Behavior

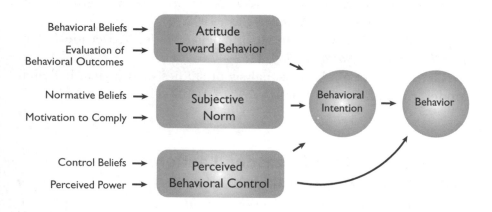

Intentions to act are thus jointly determined by attitudes and subjective norms. Put simply, the theory predicts that a person is most likely to intend to adopt, maintain or change a behaviour if that person believes the behaviour will benefit their health, is socially desirable, and feels social pressure to behave in that way. According to the theory, if these beliefs and social pressures are strong enough, this intention to behave will subsequently be transferred into behaviour.

Ajzen and Fishbein take this analysis a step further by indicating that it is the short-term consequences of behaviours that are the most powerful in predicting attitudes towards behaviour, and that subjective norms are most effected by significant others. These significant others might include, for example, a person's valued peers, and media celebrities and sports stars who act as role models.

Ajzen and others have developed this theory further and have added perceived behavioural control as a third influence on behavioural intentions. This recognises that a person's intentions will become significantly greater if they feel they have greater personal control over a behaviour — a concept closely allied to self-efficacy — and that this is also mediated by their perceived power in relation to a given situation. In making this adjustment Ajzen recognised that there are many factors beyond the immediate control of individuals which will shape their ability to behave in a desired way. As a consequence Ajzen proposed changing the name of the theory to theory of planned behaviour.

The theory can be very useful in thinking about what information you may need to collect from a target group before a program is developed. It highlights the need to understand the beliefs of the group about the issue, whom they see as affecting these beliefs and their behaviour, and what they see as the barriers to taking actions that might promote their health.

For example, in developing a diabetes education program in a community of recently arrived migrants it will be important to understand what they believe are the causes of diabetes and the actions that they feel they can confidently take to reduce their risk. It will also be important to identify who the significant others are in shaping decisions that could reduce the risk of diabetes. If the program was trying to change eating patterns it may be the oldest woman in the household or the eldest son who has most influence over the family's diet.

Ajzen and Fishbein's original model was widely applied to the development of programs to reduce uptake of smoking among youth during the 1980s. These programs recognised that information on the consequences of smoking should emphasise the short-term negative consequences (for example, on appearance, and the financial cost), as opposed to long-term negative consequences such as lung cancer and heart disease. Such programs also recognised the role of significant others in shaping decisions to smoke, by utilising peer leaders in smoking education programs, and by recruiting acknowledged role models for young people. The results of these programs were weaker than expected and led to further refinement of the theory.

Commentary

Applications of the model have demonstrated its usefulness in identifying factors which influence health behaviour that may become targets for intervention. Past failures of programs based on the theory of reasoned action have not only highlighted the difficulty of translating models which predict behaviour change into successful health promotion interventions, but also the dangers of choosing to focus on one or few elements in a complex model. The model is most successfully applied when all elements are considered in an intervention. As with the health belief model, the theory of reasoned action provides valuable insight into key factors which influence behaviour, and provides a strong indication of the importance of perceived social norms, and understanding of short-term consequences in shaping health behaviour.

Further reading

Ajzen I, Fishbein M. *Understanding Attitudes and Predicting Social Behaviour.* Englewood Cliffs, NJ: Prentice-Hall, 1980.

Ajzen I. The Theory of Planned Behaviour. *Organizational Behaviour and Human Decision Processes.* 1991; 50: 179–211.

Montano DE, Kasprzyk D, Taplin SH. The Theory of Reasoned Action and Theory of Planned Behaviour. In Glanz K et al. *Health Behaviour and Health Education: Theory, Research and Practice.* San Francisco, CA: Jossey-Bass, 1997.

2.3 The transtheoretical (stages of change) model

This model was developed by Prochaska and DiClamente to describe and explain different stages of change which appear to be common to most behaviour change processes. The model has two basic dimensions which describe both the different stages of change, and processes of change relevant to the different stage. The model is based on the premise that behaviour change is a process, not an event, and that individuals have varying levels of motivation, or readiness to change.

Five basic stages of change have been identified:
- **precontemplation:** this describes individuals who are not even considering changing behaviour, or are consciously intending not to change;

- **contemplation:** the stage at which a person considers making a change to a specific behaviour;
- **determination, or preparation:** the stage at which a person makes a serious commitment to change;
- **action:** the stage at which behaviour change is initiated; and,
- **maintenance:** sustaining the change, and achievement of predictable health gains. Relapse may also be the fifth stage.

A sixth stage of termination has also been identified as appropriate to some behaviours, especially addictive behaviours. This represents a stage where individuals have no temptation and high self-efficacy in relation to the changed behaviour, as though they had never acquired the habit (such as smoking) in the first place.

People appear to move in a predictable way through these stages, although some move more quickly than others, and some get 'stuck' at a particular stage. The model is circular rather than linear, as people can enter or exit at any point, and it applies equally to people who self-initiate change, and those who are responding to advice from health professionals, or to health campaigns.

This model has application at both the individual and broader program level. For example, for health practitioners, such as general practitioners, this model provides a useful way of thinking about the advice that they are trying to give patients and may help to reduce the frustration they feel when their advice is not taken. The model provides a way of establishing if their patient wants to change, assists in identifying barriers to making change, and recognises that relapsing is a common problem in any change process (see table 3).

From a program planning perspective, the model is particularly useful in indicating how different processes of change can influence how programs or activities are staged. Prochaska and colleagues have identified several processes of change which have been most consistently useful in supporting movement between stages. These different processes are more or less applicable at different stages of change. By matching stages of behavioural change with specific processes the model specifies how interventions could be organised for different populations with different needs and in different circumstances. The stages of change model provides important advice on the need to research the characteristics of the target population (not to assume that all people are at the same stage) and the need to organise interventions sequentially to address the different stages that will be encountered.

Commentary

The transtheoretical model has quickly become an important reference point in health interventions on a range of issues including smoking cessation, physical activity, weight control, and use of mammography services. Apart from the obvious advantage in health promotion of focussing on the change process, the model is important in emphasising the range of needs for intervention in any given population, and the changing needs of different populations. It illustrates the importance of tailoring programs to the real needs and circumstances of individuals, rather than assuming an intervention will be equally applicable to all.

Although the transtheoretical model has been proposed as a model which serves as an umbrella for other theories which guide health promotion practice, its strong roots in behavioural psychology and primary application in clinical settings with individuals makes this assessment somewhat optimistic. It may be best considered as an approach to defining health promotion needs for individuals or groups.

Further reading

Prochaska JO, DiClimente CC. The transtheoretical approach: Crossing traditional boundaries of therapy. Homewood Ill: Dow Jones Irwin, 1984.

Prochaska JO, Redding CA, Evers KE. The transtheoretical model and stages of change. In: Glanz K et al. *Health Behaviour and Health Education: Theory, Research and Practice.* San Francisco, CA: Jossey-Bass, 1997.

Prochaska JO et al. Stages of Change and Decisional Balance for Twelve Problem Behaviors. Health Psychology 1994; 13: 39–51.

2.4 Social learning theory

Social learning theory is widely considered to be the most complete theory currently applied to health promotion because it addresses both

TABLE 3: Use of the transtheoretical model by general practitioners to promote weight control among patients

Stages of change	Issue	GP action
Precontemplation	Awareness-raising	Discusses with the patient the health problems associated with being overweight
Contemplation	Recognition of the benefits of change	Discusses with the patient the potential benefits to them of proposed change
Determination or preparation	Identification of barriers	Assists patient in identifying potential barriers they may face and how these can be addressed
Action	Program of change	Works out a plan for weight loss and exercise with the patient and monitors closely
Maintenance	Follow-up	Organises for routine follow-up and discusses with patient the likelihood of relapse

the underlying determinants of health behaviour, and methods of promoting change. Social learning theory has evolved with input from several researchers over the past 50 years but, in terms of its application to health promotion, the most influential writer has been Albert Bandura. The major elements of the theory are indicated in italics. Refer to the further reading for a full and more detailed explanation.

Social learning theory was built on an understanding of the interaction which occurs between an individual and their environment. Early psycho-social research tended to focus on the way in which an environment shapes behaviour, by making it more or less rewarding to behave in particular ways. For example if at work there is no regulation on where people are able to smoke cigarettes, it is easy to be a smoker, if regulations are in place it is more difficult and most smokers smoke less and find such an environment more supportive for quitting.

Social learning theory indicates that the relationship between people and their environment is subtle and complex. For example, in circumstances where a significant number of people are nonsmokers, and are assertive about their desire to restrict smoking in a given environment, even without formal regulation, it becomes far less rewarding for the individual who smokes. They are then likely to modify their behaviour. In this case the nonsmokers have influenced the smoker's perception of the environment (referred to as *situation*) through social influence.

Bandura refers to this principal as *reciprocal determinism*. It describes the way in which behaviour and environment continuously interact and influence each other. Understanding of this interaction, and the way in which (in the example) modification of social norms can impact on behaviour, offers an important insight into how behaviour can be modified through health promotion interventions. For example, seeking to modify social norms regarding smoking is considered to be one of the most powerful ways of promoting cessation among adults.

Added to this basic understanding of the relationship between behaviour and the environment, Bandura has also determined that a range of personal cognitive factors form a third part to this relationship, affecting and being affected by specific behaviours and environments. Of these cognitions, three are particularly important. First is the capacity to learn by observing both the behaviour of others, and the rewards received for different patterns of behaviours *(observational learning)*. For example some young women may observe behaviours such as smoking by people whom they regard as sophisticated and attractive (role models). If they observe and value the rewards that they associate with smoking, such as sexual attractiveness, or a desirable self-image, then they are more likely to smoke themselves — their *expectancies* in relation to smoking are positive. Such an understanding further reinforces the importance of taking account of peer influences and social norms on health behaviour, and of the potential use of role models in influencing social norms.

Second is the capacity to anticipate and place value on the outcome of different behaviour patterns (referred to as *expectations*). For example if you believe that smoking will help you lose weight, and place great value on losing weight then you are more likely to take up or to continue smoking. This understanding emphasises the importance of understanding personal beliefs and motivations underlying different behaviours, and the need to emphasise short-term and tangible benefits or negative effects of behaviours. For example, young people have been shown to respond far more negatively to the short-term effects of smoking (bad breath, smelly clothes) than to any long-term threat posed to health by lung cancer or heart disease.

Thirdly, Bandura's work emphasises the importance of belief in your own ability to successfully perform a behaviour (referred to as *self-efficacy*). Self-efficacy is proposed as the most important prerequisite for behaviour change, and will affect how much effort is put into a task and the outcome of that task. The promotion of self-efficacy is thus an important task in the achievement of behaviour change, and Bandura has proposed that both observational learning, and participatory learning (e.g. by supervised practice and repetition) will lead to the development of the knowledge and skills necessary for behaviour change *(behavioural capability)* and are powerful tools in building self-confidence and self-efficacy.

As is the case in the interaction between behaviour and the environment, the relationship between these personal characteristics, behaviour and the environment is reciprocal and dynamic. For example, a young woman who is quitting smoking may be very confident (high self efficacy) in her ability to abstain at work where smoking is banned and none of her workmates smoke, but she may be less confident when she goes out with her friends who are heavy smokers. Thus, self-efficacy is both behaviour-specific and situation- (environment) specific.

This explicit acknowledgment of the dynamic and reciprocal relationship between an individual, their behaviour, and the environment avoids overly simple solutions to health problems which focus on behaviour in isolation from the social environment. An understanding of the characteristics of the person assists in the creation of educational interventions to alter the knowledge, understanding, beliefs and skills which affect observational learning, outcome expectations and self-efficacy. Such interventions are intended to improve the capacity of an individual to behave in a desired way. Understanding the way in which the physical and social environments act to provide incentives or disincentives for different behaviours points to ways of constructing interventions to modify the environment to further support healthy behaviours, and provide opportunities to change. Recognition that the importance of factors relating to the person and the environment will vary with different behaviours adds a further depth to the development of an intervention.

Commentary

Taken as a whole, social learning theory provides insight into approaches to improve the knowledge and skills of individuals to act to improve their health. It also explicitly identifies the importance of social norms and cues, and environmental influences on health behaviour, and again provides practical direction on how to modify these influences. In this sense it provides an important bridge between this section of the monograph and the sections which follow on community mobilisation, organisational change and public policy development.

The model also suggests a role for the health practitioner which may be less overtly interventionist in the way implied by the models described earlier. The health worker becomes a 'change agent', facilitating change through modification of the social environment and the development of personal competencies which enable individuals to act to improve their health.

It also assists in understanding the levels or layers at which a health promotion program may need to work. For example, in trying to reduce the number of young women who take up smoking it may be as important to address the issue of body image as to provide information on the short- and long-term consequences of smoking.

Not surprisingly, a review of health promotion literature in the past decade reveals a large number of health promotion interventions which combine educational programs with modification of the social and phys- ical environments based on social learning theory. This continuous 'field testing' adds further confidence in the usefulness of this theory to guide practice.

Further reading

Bandura A. *Social Foundations of Thought and Action: A Social Cognitive Theory.* Englewood Cliffs, NJ: Prentice Hall, 1986.

Bandura A. *Self-Efficacy in Changing Societies.* New York: Cambridge University Press, 1995.

Baranowski T, Perry CL, Parcel G. How Individuals, Environments and Health Behaviour Interact. In: Glanz K et al. *Health Behaviour and Health Education: Theory, Research and Practice.* San Francisco, CA: Jossey-Bass, 1997.

2.5 Summary

This overview of key theories that explain health behaviour and health behaviour change by focussing on the individual provides important guidance on key elements of health promotion programs. Taken together the theories and models described above emphasise:

- The importance of *knowledge* and *beliefs* about health. All of the theories and models presented in this chapter imply a central role for health education, and refer to individual knowledge about health, emphasising the importance of personalising health information, such that it is more immediately relevant to an individual, and emphasising the short-term consequences of behaviours.

- The importance of *self-efficacy:* the belief in one's competency to take action. The development of personal skills and self-confidence which relate to self-efficacy, through such techniques as observation, supervised practice and repetition, are central to success in each of the models presented.

- The importance of *perceived social norms* and *social influences* related to the value an individual places on social approval or acceptance by different social groups. The influence of social *role models*, family and peer groups is emphasised here.

- The importance of recognising that individuals in a population may be at *different stages of change* at any one time.

- Limitations to psycho-social theories which do not adequately take account of *socio- economic and environmental conditions* which significantly shape access to services and resources.

- The importance of shaping or changing the *environment* or people's *perception of the environment* as a key element of programs.

3. Theories which explain change in communities and communal action for health

It was clear from the work of those interested in changing the behaviour of individuals that many of the factors that affect health are to be found in the communities and immediate social environments in which people live. There have been many theories and models developed to understand the ways in which communities can be mobilised to positively influence health. This section considers two aproaches which have been influential in health promotion practice, namely community mobilisation and diffusion of innovation theory.

3.1 Community mobilisation

The health behaviour research described in the previous sections focusses on the capacity of individuals to modify personal health risks. However, of equal importance is the capacity of individuals to act collectively on issues affecting their health and the health of the communities to which they belong.

Bandura's work has provided a substantial link between theories which focus on individuals and their characteristics, and the wider social and environmental context of health promotion. Health promotion has strong foundations in public health and is fundamentally directed towards improving the health of populations, and not merely of individuals. Understanding community structures, social systems, and the different organised settings in which people live their everyday lives is essential, as too is an understanding of how these structures and systems can be mobilised for health.

At a community level, several strategies for community organisation have evolved over many years. The most widely acknowledged typology to describe different approaches in health promotion is that proposed by Rothwell which distinguishes between three models of practice: locality development, social planning and social action.

Locality development emphasises community participation and ownership of issues. This approach to community mobilisation is strongly process-oriented, focussing on consensus, cooperation and building community capacity to define and solve community problems. In this model the role of a professional practitioner is as a catalyst and facilitator rather than a leader.

By contrast, social planning is more task-oriented and expert-driven. It is based on a rational–empirical approach to problem definition, and involves professional 'planners' in the development of solutions. The role of the practitioner in this model is one of 'fact gatherer and analyst' and program implementer. This model reflects epidemiological analysis of health problems, and a tightly organised, professionally determined, planned programmatic response. In reality social planners are very dependent on working with communities to identify problems and find solutions.

The third model, social action, is one which fits comfortably with modern concepts of health promotion. It is characterised by both a concern for processes which build community capacity, and with the achievement of tangible change in a community in favour of the most disadvantaged. Achieving such change inevitably involves shifts in power relationships and resources. The practitioner role in such a model is one of advocate and mediator on behalf of disadvantaged groups.

> Social action is characterised by both a concern for processes which build community capacity, and with the achievement of tangible change in a community in favour of the most disadvantaged.

In proposing these models, Rothman makes it clear that none of the models is mutually exclusive, but rather that efforts at community mobilisation will tend towards one or another of the three categorisations. The use of the term 'locality development' has been criticised because it implies that this model of community organisation is only applicable to geographically defined communities. The alternative and the more commonly used term is community development.

Meredith Minkler has contributed greatly to our understanding of the application of such models to health promotion. She identifies essential elements of community organisation for health, including the central goal of promoting community competence (having the necessary skills and leadership to be able to engage in effective problem solving), the importance of participation and 'starting where people are at', and the creation of critical consciousness among a community.

This latter element draws substantially on the writings and action of Paulo Friere who worked with illiterate and seriously disadvantaged groups in a way that helped them to better understand the political and social structures and practices which lay beneath their problems, and to develop action plans, based on critical reflection, to help change their situation. This approach to community mobilisation has been successfully adapted to solving health problems.

In each case these characteristics emphasise the centrality of the community in problem definition, planning and action to solve problems, and the establishment of structures to ensure that solutions are sustained. This emphasis is not for purely ideological reasons. Many years of practical experience of community mobilisation have shown that change is more likely to be successfully achieved and maintained when the people it affects are involved in initiating and promoting this change.

There have been many examples of ways in which local communities have been engaged in identifying and acting upon local health issues. The issues can relate to a specific location (for example, a Safe Communities Project); a particular population group (for example, indigenous populations or particular ethnic groups); or focus on a specific disease (for example, people living with HIV–AIDS or families of people with chronic mental illness). In Australia, several programs designed to minimise the spread of HIV in gay communities have both drawn on the sense of 'community' among this population, and further added to their skills and experience in acting collectively to tackle a health problem.

It is important to recognise that effective community mobilisation is built over long periods of time, has periods of high and low activity and uses a combination of approaches depending on the problem being addressed.

Commentary

Unlike the theories and models of health behaviour described in the previous sections, community mobilisation does not lend itself so comfortably to highly structured study and comprehensive theory development. It is not easy to plan or to control. In health promotion terms, the major advantages of community mobilisation as described above are in the emphasis given to tackling determinants of health, particularly in the social action model; in the principles of community participation and competency building which are at the heart of 'enabling people to exert control over the determinants of health'; and in sustaining the effects of change. At a more fundamental level, community mobilisation is directed towards achieving population-wide change in social norms and structures which will directly benefit health (for example, by improving access to services, or creating a safer environment), and indirectly to influence individual behaviours and lifestyles by changing social norms and social support. For these reasons it is a powerful component of the health promotion kitbag.

Further reading

Bracht N, editor. *Health Promotion at the Community Level.* Newbury Park, CA: Sage, 1990.

Minkler M, Wallerstein N. Improving Health through Community Organisation and Community Building. In: Glanz K et al. *Health Behaviour and Health Education: Theory, Research and Practice.* San Francisco, CA: Jossey-Bass, 1997.

Friere P. *Education for Critical Consciousness.* New York: Seabury, 1973.

Minkler M, Cox K. Creating Critical Consciousness in Health: Applications of Friere's Philosophy and Methods to the Health Care Setting. *International Journal of Health Services* 1980; 10: 311–322.

Rothman J, Tropman JE. Models of Community Organisation and Macro Practice: Their mixing and phasing. In: Cox FM, Erlich JL, Rothman J, Tropman JE, editors. *Strategies of Community Organisation* 4th edition. Itasca, Ill: Peacock, 1987.

3.2 Diffusion of innovation theory

The systematic study of the spread of new ideas in communities has its roots in the examination of how new agricultural technologies were introduced into different situations in both developed and developing countries. Subsequent investigations examined its application and relevance to the introduction of new ideas, practices and technologies in different arenas, including health. The most widely acknowledged researcher of the diffusion process in relation to health innovations is Everett Rogers who, in successive books, has synthesised experience from hundreds of case studies, and developed both the theory of innovation diffusion and its application in a wide variety of settings.

Diffusion is defined as: *the process by which an innovation is communicated through certain channels over time among members of a social system.*

An *innovation* is defined as: *an idea, practice or object perceived as new by an individual.*

In this case, it is important to emphasise the *perceived* newness of an idea, regardless of its first use or discovery. If an idea is new to an individual then it is an *innovation.*

Diffusion of innovation theory has evolved through examination of the processes by which innovations are communicated and adopted (or not). The work of Rogers and colleagues has identified five general factors which influence the success and speed with which new ideas are adopted in communities. Understanding of these factors is central to the application of diffusion theory to health promotion innovations. The factors are:

- the characteristics of the potential adopters;
- the rate of adoption;
- the nature of the social system;
- the characteristics of the innovation; and
- the characteristics of change agents.

Some individuals and groups in society tend to be quicker to pick up new ideas than others. Young people who are highly fashion conscious are both quicker to pick up and to abandon new fashions and fads than most in the community. Witness the wardrobes full of miniskirts, platform shoes, hula-hoops and yoyos! Others in the community tend to be more suspicious of change and slow to respond to 'new-fangled' ideas.

Stereotypically, farmers are cautious in their response to innovation.

Rogers uses a system of classifying different adopters into categories according to the time it takes for adoption to occur. Innovators are those 2 to 3 per cent of the population who are quickest to adopt new ideas. However, they may be regarded as fickle, and are less likely to be trusted by the majority in the community. Early adopters are those 10 to 15 per cent of the population who may be more mainstream within the community, but are the most amenable to change, and have some of the personal, social or financial resources to adopt the innovation. The early majority are those 30 to 35 per cent of the population who are amenable to change, and have become persuaded of the benefits of adopting the innovation. The late majority are those 30 to 35 per cent of the population who are sceptics and are reluctant to adopt new ideas until such time as the benefits have been clearly established. The laggards are the final 10 to 20 per cent of the population who are seen to be the most conservative, and in many cases actively resistant to the introduction of new ideas. As indicated by the different percentages for each group, Rogers suggests that their distribution in a population matches the 'normal' probability distribution curve.

From this simple classification it is possible to see how age, disposable income and exposure to the media are, for example, all important variables which will define the different types of 'adopter' and influence the speed of uptake of innovations. As ever, it is essential to know the community with whom you are working and what is likely to influence their response to new ideas.

Rogers has also proposed that the cumulative number of adopters can be plotted against time to produce the S-shaped curve shown in figure 4. Rogers emphasises that different innovations take vastly different time periods to introduce to the majority of the target population, and in some cases, will never reach the entire population. The increasing difficulty of influencing late adopters and the residual group of laggards translates into diminishing returns on effort in

FIGURE 4. The S-shaped diffusion curve and adopter categories

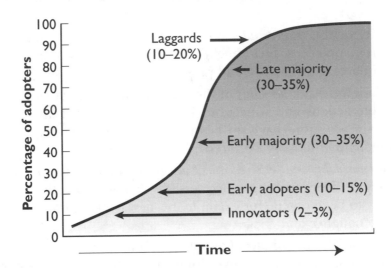

health programs, and needs to be recognised in the planning and evaluation of programs.

What becomes obvious from an examination of this model is the importance of identifying ways of speeding up the adoption process. Factors in different social systems greatly influence the rate of adoption of new ideas. 'Traditional' communities, such as rural communities in many developing countries, will generally take longer to adopt any innovation, partly because their exposure to innovations is less common, and partly because their cultures may have evolved in such a way as to be more suspicious of change.

In other social groups, change and innovation are much more common, particularly in societies with well-developed communication systems. As a consequence these populations are more experienced in dealing with innovation, and better equipped to support the process of diffusion.

Analysis of programs has led to identification of characteristics of innovations which have been consistently associated with successful adoption. These include:

- *compatibility* with prevailing socioeconomic and cultural values of the adopter (for example, the food is based on traditional food sources);

- clarity of the *relative advantage* of the innovation compared to current practices, including *perceived cost effectiveness,* as well as usefulness, convenience and prestige;

- the *simplicity and flexibility* of the innovation; those which require simple actions and which can be adapted to different circumstances are more likely to be successful (for example, no new cooking methods are required);

- the *reversibility and perceived risk* of adoption; innovations perceived as high risk or involving an irreversible change in practice are less likely to be adopted (for example, no new cooking utensils need to be bought); and

- *observability* of the results of adopting an innovation to others who may be contemplating change (for example, there are many stories in magazines showing the impact of a changed diet on a person's life).

However, it is rare for any innovation to meet all of these criteria. An understanding of these characteristics can help in the development of programs as well as in identification of implementation problems. For example, in trying to influence the diet of Aboriginal communities in remote parts of Australia it is important to recognise that more fresh food in the diet assumes that there are ways of buying, storing and cooking fresh foods, may involve more preparation time than older methods, and may require significant changes in existing food consumption patterns.

Finally, Rogers identifies the importance of the change agent who facilitates the adoption of change in a population. This may be an independent person working with a community to introduce an innovation, or may be a person from the community who is operating to facilitate change. Allied to this, community members can act as role models for other adopters. Selection of appropriate role models, particularly from among community leaders can help accelerate the rate of adoption in a community.

This latter point illustrates the coincidence of ideas between Rogers' studies of the diffusion process, and social change theory, which emphasises the central role of social modelling in learning about innovation, and in providing motivation for its adoption.

Diffusion theory is not only applicable to the introduction of new ideas into communities, but can also be considered in relation to organisations. This is of great importance in the context of health promotion, both in terms of creating supportive environments for health, and in the long-term maintenance of programs. The same type of analysis as that described above can be applied to organisations. Various studies have examined, for example, the introduction of innovations to schools and health-care settings.

Commentary

Diffusion of innovation theory has been developed and tested in a wide variety of settings, and for many different purposes. It provides an excellent diagnostic tool for analysing how and why populations respond to the introduction of new ideas, emphasising the importance of systematic research and planning to maximise chances of success. The co-incidence of themes with social learning theory further emphasises the importance of role-modelling and social reinforcement of change.

Diffusion theory is of particular importance in guiding programs which are devoted to maximising the adoption of projects which have previously been shown to be effective, and is a critical tool in promoting best practice.

However there are limitations to the theory especially in relation to the concept of laggards. It may not only be conservative attitudes and resistance to change that prevent them from adopting new behaviours, but also a lack of resources or other structural barriers. An uncritical adoption of the notion of limited returns in trying to change the remaining 20 per cent of a population may reinforce inequalities that are not necessarily due to individual choice.

Further reading

Rogers EM. *Diffusion of Innovations* 3rd edition. New York: Free Press, 1983.

Parcel GS, Perry Cl, Taylor WC. Beyond Demonstration: Diffusion of Health Promotion Innovations. In: Bracht N, editor. *Health Promotion at the Community Level.* Newbury Park, CA: Sage, 1990.

Oldenburg B, Hardcastle DM, Kok G. Diffusion of Innovations. In: Glanz K et al. *Health Behaviour and Health Education: Theory, Research and Practice.* San Francisco, CA: Jossey- Bass, 1997.

3.3 Summary

This overview of two influential approaches to achieving change in populations demonstrates the spectrum of methods in health promotion which characterise current practice. These range from those which are strongly based on building community competency and control as an integral element to achieving improvements in health, through to those which are overtly health-goal directed and which draw upon sophisticated understanding of how to speed the diffusion of predesignated ideas in communities. Each of these approaches has to be considered on its merits, and placed in the context (people, place and time) in which a program is being developed. Several key themes can be extracted from this overview:

- A focus on community action has the advantage of more overtly *addressing the social, economic and environmental determinants of health*, both directly, by achieving change in social and environmental conditions affecting health, and indirectly, by achieving population-wide change in social norms which influence behaviours and healthy lifestyles.

- Personal skills for health not only include those required to take action to modify individual behaviour, but also the *capacity to act collectively* with others to improve health.

- The diffusion of new ideas and practices through communities does not occur by chance, and can be significantly influenced by *effective change agents* in communities. The importance of effective mass communication and rolemodelling is emphasised in this process.

- Reducing inequities in health may involve investing additional resources in building the capacity of those sections of the community that are most disadvantaged.

4. Models which guide communication to bring about behaviour change

The content and form of a message can influence audience response.

As has been outlined in the previous sections, the development of effective health promotion strategies involves engaging individuals and communities in the issue. This involves an understanding of the beliefs and knowledge that people have about a problem and their skills in addressing it, as well as broader community understanding of why the issue is important and how it can most effectively be addressed.

Clear communication between health promotion practitioners and those whom they are trying to influence is essential. This communication can be at an individual level or through the development of mass communication strategies. Several models of how this can best be done have now emerged, and two of these are outlined below. They are the communication-behaviour change model and the social marketing model.

4.1 Communication-behaviour change model

The communication-behaviour change model was developed by McGuire to design and guide public education campaigns. It is included here because the model is based on communication inputs and outputs which are designed to influence attitudes and behaviour in similar ways to the models previously described.

The five communication inputs are described by McGuire:

Source: the person, group or organisation from whom a message is perceived to have come. The source can influence the credibility, clarity and relevance of a message.

Message: what is said and how it is said. The content and form of a message can influence audience response. For example the use of fear or humour to communicate the same message may provoke different responses from different target audiences. Practical considerations such as length of message, form of language and tone of voice are also included here.

Channel: the medium through which a message is delivered. These media include, television, radio, newspapers, direct mail, and more recently, electronic communication. Issues to be considered here include the potential reach of different media, the cost of use, and differences in the complexity of message which can be communicated through different media.

Receiver: the intended target audience. The gender, age, ethnic background, current attitudes and behaviours of relevance, and media use of the target population are all of importance in matching the right message to the right channel from the right source.

Destination: the desired outcome to the communication. This may include change in attitudes or beliefs, or more likely, changes in behaviour.

This model can be very useful in conceptualising and designing mass communication strategies. For example, in trying to highlight men's health issues it will be important for the source of the message to be someone respected by the men most at risk and with whom they can identify. The message will need to be portrayed in an acceptable way, for example by using humour to portray situations they face. It will need to be communicated through media used by these men with decisions made on which messages can best be communicated by TV, which by printed material, and which through advertisements. There will need to be some decision on who is the target group: is it all men? what are the subgroups? how influential are 'significant others', such as their partners and parents, in bringing about change? And finally what is it that the communication strategy is hoping to achieve; awareness raising, or some more specific action?

The communication-behaviour change model also provides a 12-step sequence of events, representing outputs from a communication, which link initial exposure to a communication to long-term change in behaviour. These are listed below:

- Exposure
- Attention
- Interest
- Understanding
- Skills acquisition

- Attitude change
- Memorisation
- Recall
- Decision-making
- Behaviour change
- Reinforcement
- Maintenance

These steps illustrate that for a communication strategy to be effective the message has to be carefully designed and delivered through an appropriate channel to reach the target audience. That population has to be exposed to the message (no mean feat in itself!), pay attention to it and understand it. Even if a message has achieved this, there are still eight more steps to the achievement of sustainable health behaviour change.

Once understood by an individual, the message must create an inclination to change, reflected in attitude change which is stored and maintained until such time as the receiver is in a position to act on that attitude change. Once the decision to change a behaviour has been made and acted on, this new behaviour needs reinforcement to be maintained.

These inputs and outputs can be put together as a matrix to illustrate the need to change the input mix depending on the targeted output. Different sources, messages and channels will be required to reach different receivers and achieve different outcomes.

Commentary

Even though this model is not based on substantial empirical testing in the same way as the health belief model and theory of reasoned action, it is based on the same general links between perceptions, attitudes and behaviour which are illustrated by these other models.

The communication-behaviour change model shows just how difficult it can be to develop a public communication campaign which by itself leads to sustainable behaviour change. This model provides an excellent overview of the range of issues which need to be considered in the development of a public education campaign. Although several major public intervention programs (such as the first Stanford three-cities program in the US, which was intended to reduce the risks for heart disease in the community) have been based on this model, progressive experience in using the mass media for public communication has led to a better understanding of the advantages and limitations of media campaigns in terms of cost, reach and effect. Media campaigns are now more commonly used to influence public knowledge, attitudes and opinions as a part of a more comprehensive strategy which places mass communication within a wider repertoire of interventions.

Further reading

Egger G, Donovan R, Spark R. Health and the Media: Principles and Practices for Health Promotion. Sydney: McGraw-Hill, 1993.

McGuire WJ. Theoretical Foundations of Campaigns. In: Rice RE, Atkin C, editors. Public Communication Campaigns. Thousand Oaks, CA: Sage, 1989.

Atkin C, Wallack L. Mass Communication and Public Health. Newbury Park, CA: Sage, 1990.

4.2 Social marketing

Social marketing evolved as a technique to influence social norms and health behaviours in the 1970s. These early approaches were based on the simple adaptation of established commercial marketing techniques for the achievement of social change. More recently, social marketing has been defined as:

> The application of commercial marketing technologies to the analysis, planning, execution and evaluation of programs designed to influence the voluntary behaviour of target audiences in order to improve their personal welfare and that of society.[2]

This definition emphasises the importance of benefit to individuals and society. It is these benefits and the nature of the relationship between the 'buyer' (communities and priority populations) and 'seller' (health promotion practitioner) that helps to distinguish social marketing for health promotion and disease prevention from commercial marketing.

In commerce, marketing is designed to influence consumer choice. The marketplace exchange is the commodity or service sold, and money collected. Success can be measured in the volume of these exchanges. Although improving knowledge of a product, or changing attitudes and values towards the product may be a means to influence purchasing behaviour, these are not in themselves the objective of marketing.

Social marketing is also intended to influence how people think and, ultimately, how they behave. Similarly it is based on a change in behaviour with costs and benefits to the individuals concerned. Immunisation offers protection against measles; a parent considers the costs and benefits of this 'product', and decides whether or not to engage in this behaviour — whether to 'buy' immunisation. Success can be measured in the number of people who are immunised.

Although the costs may not be financial, and the benefit not material, the same objective of achieving a change in behaviour is at the heart of the social marketing process. However, social marketing does differ from commercial marketing in its intent to benefit the target population and/or society in general, rather than to benefit the marketer. Thus the relationship between the 'seller' and 'buyer' will in many cases be very different from that in commercial marketing.

The planning and execution of social marketing strategies is based on a sequence of steps similar to the planning and evaluation cycle illustrated in Fiure 1 on page 10. These account for the needs of the target audience, the development and implementation of a marketing strategy to reflect those needs, and tracking of audience response to the strategy.

Market analysis

Social marketing has a strong 'consumer' orientation, rather than a focus on selling a product or service through persuasive communication. This requires a good understanding of the priority population through market research into underlying knowledge and attitudes to the issue or service, and potential channels for communication (e.g.

[2] Andreasen AR. Marketing Social Change: Changing Behaviour to Promote Health, Social Development, and the Environment. San Francisco, CA: Jossey-Bass, 1995.

literacy, media use). Such market research is intended to lead to clearly defined marketing objectives and strategies for achieving them, and to allow for segmentation of different priority populations with different needs and interests. This is followed by development and testing of the marketing plan elements, and subsequent implementation, for example, finding out the groups of people in which immunisation rates are lowest and their reasons for not immunising their children.

> Social marketing differs from commercial marketing in its intent to benefit the target population and/or society in general, rather than to benefit the marketer.

Selecting channels and materials: the marketing mix

Marketing strategies are multifactorial and generally based on achieving a balanced mix of four major inputs, commonly referred to as the four Ps of product, price, promotion and placement.

The *product* is often difficult to define in a health promotion program; we are not often selling tangible goods or services, or immediate rewards for expenditure. Identifying what is 'on offer', and presenting an appropriate image for the priority population is essential. For example, in the case of immunising children it is important to distinguish between the procedure (the injection), the service offered (the visit to GP or nurse), and the health status achieved (protection against future disease) as each may have different meaning and relevance to different target populations.

The *price* signifies the relationship between the costs and benefits of the 'product'. The costs may be real or perceived, and may include financial (e.g. the cost of visiting the GP), social (e.g. social pressure from family to have the child immunised), or opportunity costs (e.g. taking time off work to attend a local clinic). Equally, the benefits may be real or perceived. The costs and benefits of advocated actions need to be carefully considered in relation to different population subgroups. In the case of immunisation, many parents may never have seen a child with a vaccine-preventable disease and have no real conception of what it is they are trying to prevent. Strategies to effectively communicate benefits, and to reduce costs, (real and perceived) have to be developed. Such an analysis is similar to the analysis of benefits and barriers described in the health belief model.

A wide range of techniques for promotion are used in social marketing. These include the purchased media (e.g. advertising, leaflets), nonpurchased media (e.g. news coverage), sponsorship, participation events, direct selling, competitions and so on. Selecting the most appropriate channel, message delivery and source for the priority population are essential for success. Such an analysis could be based on the development of inputs described by McGuire in his communication-behaviour change model.

In all forms of marketing the final step to success is in finding high access points for a defined priority population: the right placement. This critical aspect of 'access' has often been neglected in the development of health programs. For example, the use of health screening services is determined in part by the convenience of access, and the sensitivity of service providers to language barriers, different cultural and religious norms.

Achieving the right marketing mix is at the heart of the social marketing process. Failure to address any one of the four elements will reduce the chances of success, as will over-concentration on one element alone. There can be nothing more frustrating than, for example, mounting a successful campaign to promote uptake of immunisation, only to find that service providers are unable to cope with increased demands for services, and stocks of vaccine are running low.

Implementation, assessment and feedback

These stages represent the management of a social marketing program, and are not unique to social marketing in that sense. Monitoring the implementation of a program according to a planned schedule, and monitoring its impact and effects according to predetermined objectives are a routine element to all health promotion programs. Social marketing is an iterative process, and the model is intended to account for changes in audience responses and changes in the external environment which governs the implementation process (e.g. funding and organisational structures). In this final stage, any changes to the environment are considered alongside information from the evaluation to guide the evolution of the next cycle.

Commentary

Social marketing offers a sophisticated model for achieving defined behavioural objectives in identified priority populations. It is less a theory in the formal sense defined earlier, than a planning model for health promotion. The social marketing wheel illustrates the cyclical nature of the marketing process, offering a systematic, research-based process for problem solving which includes the planning, implementation and feedback loops which are common to such models. It offers an opportunity to integrate elements of different theories (such as the health belief model, and the communication-behaviour change model), using each to advantage in a complete program model.

It is particularly useful because it encourages creative approaches to the analysis of issues and the development of programs, especially in relation to the development of channels for communication and messages. For example, social marketing has encouraged us to look outside of typical analyses of populations (e.g. age, sex, social class) in order to define consumer groups based on their media consumption or family structure, for example. Social marketing has supported experimentation with the use of a wide repertoire of different intervention methods including mass communication, sponsorship of events, and competitions, all of which have been effectively used for health promotion. Social marketing also supports a strong consumer focus in the development and delivery of programs.

However, it would be a mistake to imagine that social marketing simply involves taking marketing strategies from the commercial sector and applying them to achieve health goals. The 'product' in terms of improved health or protection against disease is often intangible, the 'price' usually not financial. Health promotion programs also operate from a different philosophical and moral base from many traditional marketing campaigns which are driven by financial gain. In such circumstances the marketing techniques to achieve sustained mass behaviour change are a great deal more complex than promoting a tangible product based on financial exchange in the commercial marketplace.

Further reading

Andreasen AR. Marketing Social Change: Changing Behaviour to Promote Health, Social Development, and the Environment. San Francisco, CA: Jossey-Bass, 1995.

Kotler P, Roberto EL. Social Marketing: Strategies for Changing Public Behaviour. New York: Free Press, 1989.

Ling JC, Franklin BA, Lingstead JF, Gearon AN. Social Marketing: Its Place in Public Health. *Annual Review of Public Health 1992*; 13: 341–62.

4.3 Summary

Both of the models presented in this section provide insight and guidance on the strengths and weaknesses of mass communication for health promotion. The social marketing theory provides a substantial model for planning and executing an integrated mass communication campaign.

Both models illustrate the limits of different forms of mass communication in producing substantial mass behaviour change, but also illustrate the important role of mass communication in raising awareness of health issues, and in securing public and political support for different forms of health promotion intervention. Both models indicate the complexity of mass communication, and illustrate:

- the importance of a*dequate market research* to define issues, segment target populations and to test communication ideas;

- the need to *match the source, message, medium and receiver* in developing mass communication campaigns;

- the need to consider a *wide range of different methods* of communication, and *different venues and settings* (promotion and placement) in the development of mass communication campaigns; and

- the importance of basing the evaluation of mass communication campaigns on *realistically defined outcomes.*

5. Models which explain change in organisations and the creation of health-supportive organisational practice

Health promotion practitioners are interested in influencing organisations for a number of reasons:

- they are usually employed by organisations and have an interest in ensuring that their own organisation is able to support the work that they are doing;
- often they are interested in influencing the activities or policies of other organisations who have an influence on the health of the population; and
- there is increased interest in finding ways to facilitate organisations working together to promote the health of the population.

Goodman, Steckler and Kegler have succinctly described the problems and potential rewards of facilitating change in organisations:

> Organisations are layered. Their strata range from the surrounding environment at the broadest level, to the overall organisational structure, to the management within, to work groups, to each individual member. Change may be influenced at each of these strata, and health promotion strategies that are directed at several layers simultaneously may be most durable in producing the desired results. The health professional who understands the ecology of organisations and who can apply appropriate strategies has a powerful tool for change.

Unlike many of the theories and models described above, the application to health problems of existing theories concerning organisational change is far less developed and analysed, and much less systematically tested in the area of health promotion. Two approaches to organisational change are considered, both are based on systematic observation of practice, combined with analysis of existing theory.

5.1 Theories of organisational change

Most of our understanding of how to produce organisational change has come from the development of management theory (and practice). This body of theory and knowledge has developed to explain organisational change for a variety of purposes, often in relation to improving organisational performance. This literature provides useful clues as to how to analyse different organisational settings, and how to plan for change.

The health professional who understands the ecology of organisations and who can apply appropriate strategies has a powerful tool for change.

Goodman, Steckler and Kegler propose a four-stage model for organisational change which appears to be applicable to health promotion practice. They emphasise the importance of recognising the different stages, and of matching strategies to promote change in each of the stages, similar to the stages of change theory, and diffusion of innovation theory.

In the model, stage 1 is described as *awareness raising*. This stage is intended to stimulate interest and support for organisational change at a senior level by clarifying health-related problems in the organisational environment, and identifying potential solutions. For example, awareness raising may involve senior managers and administrators in the education system becoming concerned about tobacco control and recognising the potential role to be played by the education system. These 'senior level administrators' are likely to be the most influential in decisions to adopt new policies and programs in an organisation. If they are convinced of the importance of a problem and the need for a solution involving their organisation, then the strategy moves to the next stage.

Stage 2 is described as *adoption,* and involves planning for and adoption of a policy, program or other innovation which addresses the problem identified in stage 1. This includes the identification of resources necessary for implementation. In larger organisations, this stage will often involve a different level in the management structure

— the 'gatekeepers' — who are more closely associated with the day-to-day running of an organisation. In the example this could involve school principals and senior teachers responsible for school curricula and organisation. Ideally, this stage will involve negotiation and adaptation of intervention ideas in order to make them compatible with the circumstances of individual organisations. This element of adaptation is often essential to the adoption of change in organisations, but frequently missed by those attempting to disseminate new ideas through organisations.

Stage 3 is described as *implementation,* and is concerned with technical aspects of program delivery, including the provision of training and material support needed for the introduction of change. In the example, this could involve classroom teachers, as they will be most directly responsible for the introduction of change. This phase may involve training and the provision of resource support to foster the successful introduction of a program. This capacity building is essential for the successful introduction and maintenance of change in organisations. Many policy initiatives fail at this point because too little attention is given to the detail of the implementation process, and too little support is offered to the individuals at the level at which implementation takes place in an organisation.

Stage 4 is described as *institutionalisation* which is concerned with the long-term maintenance of an innovation, once it has been successfully introduced. Senior administrators again become the leading players, by establishing systems for monitoring and quality control, including continued investment in resources and training.

Commentary

This model is particularly helpful in illustrating the ways in which organisations function at different levels, how the achievement of organisational change may be achieved in a staged process, and how each stage may require involvement of different levels in an organisation. The model is most useful in situations where an organisation is viewed as a potential host institution to previously developed health programs. It does not so easily accommodate health promotion strategies which seek to help organisations to develop in a more holistic way, such as to develop organisational policy and practices as a means to creating safe and health supportive environments for workers and clients.

Further reading

Goodman RM, Steckler A, Kegler MC. Mobilising Organisations for Health Enhancement: Theories of organisational change. In: Glanz K et al. *Health Behaviour and Health Education: Theory, Research and Practice.* San Francisco, CA: Jossey-Bass, 1997.

5.2 A model of intersectoral action

As well as working with organisations as potential host institutions for existing programs, and as a means to creating supportive environments for health, we need increasingly to work with organisations as partners in the development and implementation of health promotion programs. There are no theories or models which define this process of intersectoral action but there have been several attempts to review experience in intersectoral action, and in related activities such as coalition-building in the recent past. These reviews have identified different sets of factors that are important to understanding the process by which organisations, or parts of organisations, work together. These include:

- *an understanding of the context:* the reasons why organisations need to work together, and an analysis of the opportunities that exist in their organisational environments that will support action.

- *an assessment of the infrastructure:* whether the organisations have the capacity to undertake the planned action, and the nature of the relationship required to take agreed actions.

- *a planned approach to action and sustainability:* a plan of action that has benefits for all involved, and clarifies the different roles and relationships required to take action.

A review undertaken by the authors and colleagues of intersectoral action in Australia has proposed a framework for understanding the factors that will influence effective intersectoral action. In this model six factors were identified as important dimensions to effective inter-

Successful collaboration between organisations needs to build on the foundations of necessity and opportunity.

sectoral action: the necessity for the sectors or organisations to work together; the factors that are providing the opportunity for them to work together; the capacity to work together; established relationships that will allow them to achieve their goal; the action they are undertaking should be planned and able to be evaluated; and the action should be sustainable.

Understanding the context

Successful collaboration between organisations needs to build on the foundations of *necessity* and *opportunity*. Organisations are more likely to be open to collaboration and change if it helps them to *pursue core business more effectively or efficiently*. This core business may have nothing to do with health in a direct sense, but may have an indirect impact on health , for example if the core business is transport or housing programs, or the activities of private sector companies promoting different foods. In addition to achieving their organisational goals, organisations are also interested in working together:

- to attract or protect resources;
- to protect or gain in their areas of influence; and
- to be seen as good corporate citizens.

Understanding the strength of the motivation for organisations to work together assists in understanding the level of commitment they will be willing to make, and of risk they will be willing to take.

The opportunity for taking action is reflected in immediate organisational priorities. These may be in response to crises within organisations, or a response to unpredicted events outside the organisation, for example a number of fatal football injuries may make it more likely that sporting organisations will be more receptive to advice concerning changes in rules recommended by the health sector in the past. However, without the infrastructure to undertake action, such opportunities to work with other organisations to achieve common goals may be missed.

Assessing the infrastructure

Many of the factors which contribute to either the success or failure of a particular activity are seen as related to the capacity of the organisations to undertake that activity. This capacity is primarily reflected in:

- the level of organisational support for the activity, (including compatible structures and decision-making processes);
- adequate levels of resources, (including time, financial resources and infrastructure); and
- a skilled workforce.

The other crucial aspect of infrastructure is the relationship that exists between the organisations involved. These relationship are generally a mix of formal and informal links, and provide the mechanism within which actions can be developed and conflicts resolved.

Without adequate infrastructure it can be difficult for organisations to sustain action over time or adapt to changing circumstances.

A planned approach to action and sustainability

Building and sustaining relationships between sectors towards common goals is a difficult task. Many of the conditions for success (or failure) are in place long before any specific action is taken and it is important to not only plan the details of the project, but also to account for the context in which it is being undertaken, and the ability of the infrastructure of the organisations to deliver. From reviews of practice, several issues have emerged as important in the implementation of a project that requires cooperation between different agencies:

- clear recognition of why it is important for the organisations to work together, including agreement on how the issue and the solution are defined, and what role they see for their respective organisations in the implementation process.
- acknowledgment that *the process is emergent and changing;* the need for flexibility in negotiation over roles and responsibilities.
- definition of a *clearly articulated and achievable goal* that is understood and valued by the different organisations involved in a project.
- *agreement on a way of working;* this may mean working on small, well-defined tasks initially to build trust and confidence in a work-

ing relationship before seeking to implement more significant changes.

- *opportunities for renegotiation* including identification of the length of time to which organisations are committed, and allowing for redefinition of tasks, roles and relationships.

- commitment to joint ownership; any sense that one partner is imposing on another invariably leads to resistance and damage to the relationship.

- *allocation of resources;* staff, space, money, information and administrative support.

The case studies in table 4 illustrate how such a comprehensive analysis can help us understand why some activities are successful and others difficult.

Commentary

This analysis complements that of the previous section by offering further insight to the conditions for successfully working with other organisational structures to promote health. In particular it highlights the need to work at different levels both within and between organisations in addressing issues of common concern.

In analysing intersectoral action it is also important to understand the vision, commitment and networks of individuals involved. It is the relationship between these three factors that makes many intersectoral projects possible, and highlights the need for longer term organisational support.

Assessment of the conditions in which a project or activity is operating (the context, infrastructure and planned action) allows us to anticipate where difficulties may arise. It gives guidance on where action can be taken to strengthen these conditions at all points in the planning cycle and in ensuring that the conditions for success are in place before the action begins.

Further reading

Harris E, Wise M, Hawe P, et al. *Working Together:* intersectoral action for health. Canberra: Australian Government Publishing Service, 1995.

Goodman RM, Steckler A, Kegler MC. Mobilising Organisations for Health Enhancement: Theories of organisational change. In: Glanz K et al. Health Behaviour and Health Education: Theory, Research and Practice. San Francisco, CA: Jossey-Bass, 1997.

Butterfoss FD, Goodman R, Wandersman A. Community coalitions for prevention and health promotion. Health Education Research 1993; 8.3: 315–330.

O'Neill M, Lemieux V, Groleau G et al. Coalition theory as a framework for understanding and implementing intersectoral health-related interventions. Health Promotion International 1997; 12(1): 79–85.

TABLE 4: Applying the model for understanding intersectoral action

CASE STUDY: The NSW Children's Services Health & Safety Committee	CASE STUDY: Access to children's services
Following an outbreak of measles in 1991 the Committee was formed to improve health and safety policies and practices in child care centres. Major service providers, unions, training bodies, Public Health Units and academics have been able to work together effectively on this issue.	The same core group of people and organisations that successfully established the Health & Safety Committee have had much more difficulty in addressing lack of access to children's services for children whose parents are on low incomes and not in the workforce.
Necessity It was clear at all levels of the child care and health sectors that they needed to work together to improve policies and practices.	**Necessity** There is not a high level of concern in either the health or child care sectors about this issue, and the ways in which both sectors could work together is not clear.
	Continued over

CASE STUDY: The NSW Children's Services Health & Safety Committee

Opportunity
The dramatic increase in the number of children in care in the past decade and concern for the children's health supported the action. The measles epidemic and growing epidemiological evidence of the risks associated with care provided strong triggers for action.

Capacity
Although specific resources for the Committee were limited there was a high level of organisational support by all involved (including a research grant) and skilled workers to undertake any action.

Relationship
Most of the organisations involved had worked together before in some way. Because the action did not require high levels of joint planning or resource allocation the relationships were able to be loose and flexible.

Action
Over the past two years the Committee has focussed on research into current policies and practices and the development of model policies.

Sustainable outcomes
It is now important for the Committee to look at ways in which it can sustain any gains they have made. This will involve more formal recognition of the Committee by both sectors and the allocation of specific resources.

CASE STUDY: Access to children's services

Opportunity
Current community concern about the provision of children's services is focussed on the needs of working parents. There are few triggers for action, no obvious policies to support action in this area, limited data on the nature and extent of the problem, and no new ways of thinking about the issue.

Capacity
The organisations and individuals involved are already stretched and, although there are high levels of organisational support, there are few resources for taking action.

Relationship
To bring together all the stakeholders in this issue new relationships will need to be formed. There is little time to identify, contact and build support.

Action
Because there is little understanding of the nature and extent of the problem and little history of working together, there is no clear plan of possible action. In this case few of the conditions for effective action are in place. Rather than invest time in developing a plan of action it would be better to look at ways of making the necessity for the action more apparent, to create an environment where action is seen as important, and to look at ways of increasing the capacity of the organisations to take action.

5.3 Summary

Although the models described above are not strictly theories according to the criteria described at the beginning of the monograph, they are based on systematic observation and analysis of organisational change, and do offer guidance on factors influencing the successful introduction and maintenance of change in organisational settings. Further, systematic testing of these ideas in planned programs will be necessary to clarify their usefulness and identify further refinements.

These models provide useful guidance on the different steps required to introduce and sustain a program in different organisational settings. In particular they highlight:

- the need to understand the core business of an organisation, and its organisational structure, determine how a health promotion program can fit within these parameters, and help achieve core business;
- the need to work with individuals at different levels in an organisation as well as between organisations;
- the inherently 'political' nature of the task of influencing senior managers;
- the importance of flexibility in negotiation with 'gatekeepers' concerning the adoption of a program;
- the need to support those individuals responsible for the delivery of a program or innovation; and
- the need to establish a system for longer term maintenance and quality control.

One of the major reasons that the health sector is interested in working with other organisational structures is to bring about systematic and lasting change that will address some of the basic determinants of health, for example safe workplaces, improved living conditions or the development of recreational facilities. Understanding how to do this most effectively has the potential to have profound impacts on health.

Models which help to understand the development of healthy public policy

The mounting evidence that factors outside the control of the health sector have a profound impact on health has resulted in increasing interest in the development of public policies which protect and promote health. For example, housing, income support, employment, education, and environmental protection policies can have both a direct and indirect impact on the health of individuals and communities.

How can the policies that impact on health be influenced? This is still a developing area of study in health promotion. This section examines three frameworks that have been proposed by people aworking in the area of health promotion for understanding the development of healthy public policy.

6.1 An ecological framework for making healthy public policy

Nancy Milio has proposed a conceptual framework through which we can develop a greater appreciation of how successful public policy to improve health is developed.

In this framework, policy development is seen as passing through discrete stages of initiation, adoption, implementation, evaluation, and reformulation. These stages are part of a continuous social and political process that is not strictly linear. *The development of healthy public policy is seen as a dynamic process and not simply the production of a policy statement.*

In this framework there are four main players who are crucial in the development of healthy public policy:

- policy holders (usually politicians and bureaucracies);
- policy influencers (who can be groups inside and outside government);
- the public (audiences, consumers, taxpayers and voters) whose

opinion will ultimately affect the adoption of the policy; and

- the media (print and electronic) that influence both the policy makers and public's understanding of, and attitude towards an issue.

Although the development of healthy public policy often appears to be driven by one or a group of influential individuals Milio argues that it is the organisations and not the individuals that lead them that should be the focus of analysis. This gives a better understanding of the motivation and resource base of those involved.

Within organisations the key stakeholders are seen as falling broadly into two groups: the policy keepers who have initiated or hold a mandate for a specific policy and moves the policy at a pace based on their interests; and the policy influencers who have an interest in the issue and may try to influence the content of the policy and the speed and way in which it is implemented. For example, the police may be seen as the policy keepers in gun regulation while the policy influencers may consist of gun lobbies, public health bodies and community coalitions.

In this model the general public is not seen as influencing the formulation of specific policies in important ways, but is seen as forming part of the climate for policy-making.

A number of key determinants of influencing policy development are identified:

- the social, economic, and political context in which action is proposed (social climate);
- the identification of parties with most influence on policy development;
- the recognition of the interests of those wishing to influence policy development (what they will win or lose, where they are willing to make compromise); and
- the capacity of those wishing to develop or influence policy to put in place strategies that will be successful in representing their interests.

The social climate in which the policy is being developed has a significant impact on the relatively few political leaders who will finally make the decision to adopt a policy. For example, in the gun control debate in Australia a number of tragic mass shootings dramatically shifted the social climate from a concern for the rights of shooters towards the broader community interest to be protected from the consequences of uncontrolled access to guns.

In this case the groups wanting tighter gun control found that their power to influence change had increased. They were better placed to put forward tough proposals for gun control in the belief that government would be unlikely to ignore broad-based support. Those groups against gun control needed to find ways to re-exert their influence and put forward arguments to the government that would counterbalance community sentiments.

Milio argues that how major stakeholders respond will be coloured by what they see as in their best long-term interests. This may differ from their public statements. Groups may choose not to influence the development of the policy but rather put their effort into opposing the implementation of the policy.

Finally, it is important to understand that key players, both within and outside government, will develop strategic plans to influence the development of policies that have a high priority. The type and effectiveness of this strategy will depend on such things as the size of the organisation, their resources, organisational age (affecting experience, contacts and credibility), authority, their closeness and importance to the policy makers, and skill in using these assets.

Developing effective information strategies will be an important part of this process, for example in the gun debate, having credible spokespersons who could provide leadership and information was an important factor in developing a climate that would support change. Milio argues that the ways in which information is used will vary. It can be less active use of information to monitor, analyse and critique policy-making; or more direct efforts in persuading, mediating or mobilising others to action. This can be directed at the policy makers themselves or past them to influence credible public figures to support the issue and/or build public support. Milio sees that the media has a central role in creating public opinion not only by what they report but also by choosing whether to say anything at all, who is allowed to speak, how much prominence an issue is given and the way the issue is framed. The role of the media becomes very important when this information is not available to policy makers or the public through experience or other sources.

Commentary

This model presents a clear picture of the groups who have a role in policy development: the policy makers, interested parties, the public and the media. It highlights the need to see policy development as a dynamic process that can be influenced at many stages by those who have something to win or lose, and by the social climate in which the policy makers are operating. How this social climate is shaped will depend very much on how the media report, or fail to report the issue.

Further reading

Milio N. Making healthy public policy: developing the science by learning the art: an ecological framework for policy studies. *Health Promotion* 1987; 2(3): 263–74.

6.2 Basic determinants of policy-making to promote health

Even the most casual observer of healthy public policy can see that there is often a poor relationship between what is known about factors that cause or could prevent illness and disability and the policies in place about these issues. Epidemiologists and other population health researchers often complain that their findings are not taken up by policy makers, while policy makers complain that there is often no relevant evidence for them to base policy on.

De Leeuw proposes that there are three determinants of policy-making that need to be understood if those interested in the development of healthy public policy are to make progress:

- the bias that stems from sets of causal, final and normative assumptions and presuppositions;
- the interest webs of groups in certain domains; and
- the power of organisations to monitor and communicate their intentions.

Assumptions

Policy makers acquire in their career and work environment a set of assumptions and beliefs about general policy directions. Three sets of assumptions that affect policy development are proposed: those around the relationship between cause and effect; those between intervention and outcome, and underlying values. Together they are seen as forming a set of assumptions and presuppositions that is the framework in which policy objectives, instruments and time frames are established and assessed. Very rarely are these assumptions and presuppositions made explicit although they set the parameters of action that will be seen as desirable and feasible.

For example, in exerting pressure for the development of policies to address the health impact of unemployment, these three sets of assumptions appear to influence the views of those involved. The relationship between unemployment (cause) and poor health (effect) is often perceived to be unclear — were the unemployed more likely to have lost their job because they were sick, or is their poorer health due to an unhealthy lifestyle rather than unemployment itself? There may be simplistic views about the nature of the interventions that may bring about changes in health outcomes, for instance that full employment will solve the problem. And despite the fact that there are far fewer jobs available than people to fill them there still seem to be views in the community that people would find a job if they really wanted to work, as reflected in keeping job-seeking diaries and so on.

Interests

The way policy is formulated and implemented is often determined by the vested interests of stakeholders or interest groups. For example, in efforts to reduce unemployment levels there are many vested interests that can range from those trying to deregulate the labour market as a way of promoting economic growth, through to unions who may be interested in seeing that their members do not lose their jobs, to welfare groups advocating better income support for people who are unemployed.

As well as wanting to see a reduction in unemployment, these groups need to ensure their own survival and spheres of influence. De Leeuw argues that they are often willing to undertake any action to ensure their survival. If action is to be taken that will protect and promote health then those developing the policies need to recognise the different and overlapping areas of interest and perceived needs. Providing health-based information by itself may not meet this need.

> The way policy is formulated and implemented is often determined by the vested interests of stakeholders or interest groups.

Power positions

The effectiveness that groups will have in exerting their power or influence is seen as closely related to their capacity to understand the policy and strategic intentions of their competitors and allies. For example, if the health sector is trying to introduce policies to reduce the impact of unemployment on health it needs to recognise that less powerful interests groups may see the health sector's interest as being a way to get more money for services, or as cost-shifting.

The perceived power of those involved informs any strategic action taken. The degree of power which groups have and their capacity to monitor the interests and plans of others and communicate their own intentions has proved highly predictive in the success organisations have in influencing policy.

De Leeuw's focus is on how epidemiological information can inform policy development to promote health. It is not enough to know or even communicate the 'truth'; attempts also need to be made to use this information in ways that will be taken up by major stakeholders. This involves understanding how they see the issue, how they think it is caused, how they think action will be effective; the nature of the stakeholders' interests and the way in which health interests may potentially benefit them; and a detailed understanding of the strategies used by those involved to achieve their organisational ends.

Commentary

The model developed by De Leeuw to understand the factors that will influence the development of healthy public policy provides a way of understanding why many attempts to promote a particular policy fail. It is not only because of the power of the groups involved or what they stand to gain or lose. Willingness to support a particular issue will also be influenced by what those involved believe to be the cause of the problem, what they feel can effectively be done to address it, and their assumptions and presuppositions about where health is created.

Further reading

De Leeuw E. Health policy, epidemiology and power: the interest web. Health Promotion International. 1993; 8(1): 49–53.

6.3 Establishing indicators of health promotion policy: a way to develop theory

In examining the factors that have an influence on health Ziglio argues that policy sectors such as agriculture, defence, income maintenance, transport, education and employment have a combined effect on people's health which is greater than the traditional health policies conceived as hospital and medical services:

Effectively moving towards health promotion therefore necessitates fundamental changes in traditional ways of formulating public policy. These changes should affect both the social and economic facets of public policy...to prevent rather than just mitigate the health-damaging effects of poverty and deprivation.

Ziglio argues that if the potential benefits of health promotion policy are to be realised there needs to be a substantial investment in research to understand the conditions favouring or impeding the formulation and implementation of health promotion practice. He sees the development of indicators of health promotion policy as representing an opportunity to analyse policy and begin to build theory. One of the areas seen as providing insight into the way healthy public policy can be understood is to examine the process through which decisions are made, and if practitioners want to influence these factors there need to be fundamental changes in the ways public policy is formulated.

Rational-deductive decision-making

A rational-deductive model of decision-making relies heavily on evidence and a commitment to making planned, rational choices that will bring about change. The policies developed through this model of decision-making are framed in terms of strategies with sequential steps and specific health promotion objectives. This would be reflected in:

- clear goals and objectives that govern the policy;
- an understanding of the decision-making powers of those involved (e.g. policy makers, organised groups, voluntary organisations);
- a clear set of criteria used to rule out possible policy alternatives; short- and long-term implementation schedules;
- policy evaluation and feedback mechanisms; and
- channels and processes for modifying policy based on evaluation and feedback.

These types of policies are often seen as inflexible and not able to respond to changing policy environments.

Incremental decision-making

In this style of policy development the aim is to arrive at policy decisions by muddling through, resulting in only marginal change. Decision makers focus only on those policy alternatives that are incrementally different from existing ones with only a restricted number of consequences being evaluated, and the problem confronting decision makers is continually refining it to make it more manageable.

The final set of priorities is obtained by a political process in which the pressure exerted by different issue groups plays the most important part in decision-making. This style of decision-making, common in most western industrialised countries, focusses on remedial or marginal change. This will be reflected in:

- understanding the interests of those with an interest in the area and the magnitude of competing goals and objectives;

- number, composition and power of vested-interest groups, lobbying and policy advocacy groups;
- the interaction between these groups and the processes and bargaining involved;
- the compromise, outcomes and short-term marginal change that results; and
- an assessment of the outcome in relation to overall health promotion objectives.

These types of policies are often seen as lacking long-term focus and being too influenced by the broader social and political contexts, and are difficult to evaluate.

Mixed-scanning style of decision-making

Finally, Ziglio argues that many countries are now interested in a mixed-scanning approach that tries to incorporate both rationalist and incremental principles. This implies that there is an underlying set of fundamental decisions that are based on a rationalist approach and are then influenced by political considerations and the interests of different groups. These incremental decisions need to be seen in the context of the broader and longer term vision of the fundamental decisions that are driving the decision-making process.

A mixed-scanning approach would be characterised by:
- policy statements which make clear the fundamental role of health promotion;
- a process of interaction between policy factors that has led to the development of this policy;
- criteria used in selecting health-promotion-related issues for further analysis;
- scanning of the process of interaction leading to policy statements and the criteria used for taking up issues; and
- analysis of how different interests are affecting the development of policy and why issues are being taken up.

These types of policies are seen as offering both the coherence and flexibility that are needed to cope with changing circumstances.

Commentary

Ziglio makes an important contribution to our understanding of the policy-making process by clearly outlining the three major ways in which decisions are currently seen to be made. This analysis, with its emphasis on the need to articulate the indicators by which a decision-making style would be evaluated, highlights the potential benefits of clearly articulating the outcomes we hope to see from any particular action. His support for a mixed-scanning approach allows us to see a possible need to balance an approach that is based on evidence and planning with one that can account for the political realities in which policy is developed.

Further reading

Ziglio E. Indicators of health promotion policy: directions for research. In: Bandura B, Kickbusch I. *Health Promotion Research. World Health Organization Regional Publications, European Series No. 37.* Copenhagen: WHO, 1993

Ziglio E. Policy-making and planning in conditions of uncertainty: the case of health promotion policy. *Edinburgh: Research Unit in Health and Behaviour Change, Working Paper No 7, 1987.*

6.4 Summary

Taken together these three approaches provide us with valuable guidance on how healthy public policy can be developed.

They stress the need to recognise that policy is not based solely on the evidence of the nature and extent of the problem and what are thought by health promotion practitioners to be effective strategies to address them.

In order to understand the process through which policy is developed it is important to recognise the major stakeholders and their interests; recognise their perceptions of the issue and their possible solutions; and understand possible areas of conflict and compromise.

Although not directly influential in policy development, the importance of public opinion and the general climate in which the organisations are operating are also highlighted as important. Influencing these opinions and environments is recognised as important in introducing new ideas and having policies adopted.

Epilogue: Theory in practice

This monograph provides only an introduction to the many different theories and models which have guided health promotion practice. In each case the different sections provide a synthesis of the different elements of the theories and the research which has guided their development, and indicates their reliability for guidance of practice. Readers who require more detailed information on the different theories should refer to the original texts cited in each section, or to other more comprehensive publications.

What will be apparent from the different sections is that the theory guiding practice in health promotion is not yet well developed. The theories concerning psycho-social determinants of health in individuals are the least complex and best tested according to traditional criteria. The different theories and models which may be useful to guide elements of programs directed to community mobilisation, organisational change and policy development are generally less well formed and far less amenable to testing through typical experimental research designs, such as randomised controlled trials. In such cases these may represent part of the art of health promotion as much as they represent the science. However, the importance of community mobilisation, and organisational and policy change for health is so great that it is essential to identify and apply our best current understanding of these issues. Research to advance our knowledge and understanding of such processes may be of the highest priority in the future.

There is no single theory or model which can adequately guide the development of a comprehensive health promotion program intended to influence the multiple determinants of health in populations. Practitioners need to use local knowledge and experience, and available research information to make judgments about community needs and the determinants of health which are most amenable to change at any particular time. In developing a comprehensive strategy to tackle a defined health priority, practitioners will be assisted by making judicious use of the theories and models described in this monograph. Multilevel interventions will generally be more powerful than single-track programs. Correspondingly, programs will need to draw on several of the theories and models described in the monograph in the development of a comprehensive strategy. If applied wisely, these theories will help guide decisions, may predict the likely outcomes, and help explain the reasons for success.

Not all practitioners have the position or capacity to operate at multiple levels. In such cases, a knowledge of the theories in this monograph will help practitioners to maximise the potential effectiveness of their interventions, and to place into perspective their efforts alongside the range of opportunities for action.

Index

The letters *f*, *n* and *t* following page numbers refer to figures, footnotes and tables respectively.